I0840912

Health Literacy Guide Talking to Your Provider and Healthy Living

Contents

\

Introduction

Welcome to my 6th book in the *Health Literacy Guide* series. This book, like all the rest of my Health Literacy Guides, is based on classes that I have been teaching for years in New York State. This book will cover the 10 basics skills that everyone needs to understand to be successful in communicating their medical provider- whether that is a medical doctor, pharmacist, chiropractor or Reiki Guru. If you are seeking health advice and medications or supplements from that person, they are acting as a medical provider for you.

The first three chapters of each book are nearly identical. They cover the same background questions: what is public health, what is health literacy, and what is health? You may notice some variations in the stories or points that I make in each area, but the vast majority of the information is the same.

I hope this will be a handy resource for you if you currently have a health concern, or as a tool for you to talk to loved ones about their health.

As a note: I am going to use the word doctor and office as the term for the provider you are interacting with. Understand that doctor in this book means anyone you are seeking medical advice from (chiropractor, nurse, physical therapist, reiki practitioner, staff at a health store) and office means anywhere you go (pharmacy, vitamin store, health food store, urgent care center, holistic healing center)

Be Healthy!

Karen

Chapter 1: What is Public Health?

"Good Afternoon, My name is Karen Laing and I am a public health educator. Does anyone know what public health is?" I use this opening line in every class I teach. Unless I am teaching in a community that hires me regularly, I am usually met by blank stares and a lot of head shaking. And why would you know what public health is? It is the hidden side of the medical system. It is the prevention piece of the US Healthcare system which works well for some, not at all for a few, and okay for most. Public health studies death, dying, and illnesses to help Americans to live as long as possible with minimum disability.

Public health has five areas of sub-specialties. The first is the research division, also known as epidemiology. These researchers are often found in state and federal health departments and they are the people who put out the contradictory test results. Take the effects of coffee: coffee is good for you, coffee is bad for you, coffee is good for you. At this moment, research shows the drink one makes from coffee beans is good for you...as long as you don't smoke cigarettes with it, dunk donuts into it, or put tons of cream and sugar into it, and if your body can handle the caffeine that naturally occurs within the coffee bean.

The coffee research is a great example of why research is often contradictory and further studies are often needed. Public health research does not want to assume anything: it needs to prove that the core issue and not anything else is responsible for the results. So when coffee was first deemed bad for you, people had not looked closely at the research taking out the effects of having a cigarette with your coffee. Cigarettes have been proven over and over again to be horrible little sticks of destruction, and once the results separated out the coffee-only addict vs the coffee-and-cigarette addict, coffee seemed healthier. When studies separated out those who drank coffee but paired it with highly un-nutritious food (like donuts and desserts), coffee again improved in the health realm. And again there was a difference between those who drank their coffee black, those who only used a little flavoring, and those who liked "a little coffee with their cream and sugar."

Then finally, health research goes to an individual level. Some of the most recent reports are showing extremely positive results from drinking coffee like less depression, better long-term memory, less skin cancer, liver disease and gout. Then, of course, there is the question, how does your body process the caffeine? If you cannot handle caffeine, then coffee might be just fine for your neighbor and no good for you. Just like strawberries are great, unless you are allergic to them, then you should not eat them.

Once the statisticians in the research field are pretty sure they can link a cause and effect together, they will often send the research to the second division- public policy. This is where that research goes to creating laws to keep us safe. Adding fluoride to drinking water and seat belt laws are two of America's most well-known public health policies or laws.

The environmental health section, the third division, made a huge impact in the clean air and water acts from the 60s and 70s as well as more recently with fracking and Legionnaire's disease prevention. While I was editing my first book, Hurricane Harvey hit

Houston. Houston is a city known for very few grassy areas (green space as it is called in public health.) Environmental health was already aware that the more green space there is, the healthier residents and employees tended to be. Perhaps because nature has a calming effect on people, perhaps because there is extra oxygen in the atmosphere from the plants. With very little green space in Houston, there was nowhere for the water to go to. It took longer for the water to recede and evaporate. I am sure the environmental public health division will be closely studying the effects on the buildings and residents' health when the water floods a building and city for two months in comparison to the areas around Houston that had the same intensive rain, but had green space for the water to be absorbed into the ground. My guess- look for public policy to start changing laws about the amount of green space needed for building in a year or so (the end of 2018.)

Biotechnology is the fourth subdivision of public health. Current technology is studied and continuously improved. Oxygen tanks that were highly combustible, heavy and limiting to how far a person could go with it were replaced with oxygen concentrators that are lighter weight, have little risk of exploding and simply need to be plugged in to work. The lighter weight equipment and the increased safety have greatly improved the daily lives of those who need extra oxygen to live. Again, one can see the public health focus toward allowing people to live as full a life as possible despite their chronic illnesses.

Finally, I come to the last specialty area—social, behavioral and community health. How does public health change a large society to live healthier lives? One of the ways public health does this is through vaccine clinics in stores that make it convenient for people to be vaccinated. Or through public health educators who run trainings to help people understand their illnesses better. Since I started this book with the comment, I am a public health educator; you can see that this is my specialty. I train, less on specific diseases, but on a set of core values called "Health Literacy."

Chapter 2: What is Health Literacy?

According to the US government health literacy is "the degree to which individuals have the capacity to obtain, process, and understand basic health information and services needed to make appropriate health decisions." In other words, it is a core set of skills you need to navigate the healthcare system (in sickness and in health), make healthy decisions at home, and (I have included) respond in a public health emergency. Health Literacy is understanding the ABCs of the healthcare system. Most public health educators teach on specific diseases, I teach on skills and knowledge that underlie a person's understanding of those diseases and their treatments.

Health literacy, like financial literacy, is a concept we are just beginning to recognize as key to a successful long life. If you don't know the basics of balancing a checkbook, you are inevitably going to bounce some checks along the way. If you don't understand the how and whys of taking medications (for example), you will make mistakes and end up potentially harming yourself or others.

In the United States, it is estimated that only 1 out of 10 Americans is proficient in health literacy skills. And when the mental health system is involved, the numbers go down to 1 out of 33 patients. The US medical system first recognized that patients were not fully health literate in the 1980s. Back then AIDS patients and breast cancer patients both began demanding the right to be involved in their own care. They wanted to make decisions about treatment and lifestyle choices and when to end treatment. As doctors handed patients over the right to make decisions, they realized that not all patients could make the right decisions. Medical schools responded to low health literacy by teaching doctors to use "plain language," foreign language translators and to provide education guides with pictures. While this was a good step toward better communication, it did not solve a patient's ability to ask questions and feel competent to make decisions. It changed the doctor's way of communicating, but did not improve the health literacy skills of the patients.

In 2012, I studied health literacy for a college internship. I was asked to design a tool to help a poverty-based agency screen which of its' clients needed training in health literacy. It did not take long to realize that since only 1 in 10 people were health literate, the answer was not to screen, but to train everyone. I then researched what was available to train on health literacy skills. Since it was 20 plus years since the US had identified the problem, I thought it would be easy to put together some trainings for the everyday patient to use based on what was already out in the medical community. Sadly, that was not the case. The public health sector was still fighting over whether health literacy included skills or knowledge, as well as how to assess patients' abilities to navigate.

As a retail trainer for years and a special education teacher to start my career, it made more sense to me to start training people and see how that improved health literacy skills. And so I created the first health literacy training program in the country designed to teach everyone on these basic skills. I used the bits of curriculum I could find from cancer, heart disease, and diabetes education, along with my training as a researcher to read through the latest research. I wanted to find the pieces of knowledge and define the communication aspects that would help patients clearly share with their doctors about their health concerns, needs, and values.

When I started my work, only California had a program that taught directly to patients, and they only taught low income parents who used Medicaid. By the time I was done with my internship, Florida also developed a program under its English as a Second Language program. A year later, Minnesota began teaching health literacy to seniors. To the best of my knowledge, we are the only four programs focused on teaching skills directly to patients anywhere in the world, even now six years after I started researching this issue. The rest of the country and the world are still trying to correct a patient deficit by retraining medical providers. In 2016, the agency I opened won an Award from the New York State Public Health

Association for Outstanding Leadership in Public Health for our work as Health Literacy advocates and trainers.

So how crucial is it that people have good health literacy skills? According to the federal report *Inadequate Health Literacy A Barrier to Patient Care*, patients who do not have good healthcare skills struggle unnecessarily and at a high cost. They are

1. More likely to report poor health status
2. Twice as likely to be hospitalized
3. Remain in the hospital more days per each admission
4. Have one more outpatient visit per year
5. Have more difficulty using metered inhalers
6. Have worse HbA1c levels (blood sugar levels)
7. More likely to make medication errors
8. Less likely to comply with recommended treatments.

As a result, they are more likely to be seriously disabled or die at an earlier age than someone with excellent health literacy skills. According to the National Action Plan to Improve Health Literacy, lack of health literacy skills costs the United State between $106 and $236 billion annually in medical bills alone, and an additional $238 billion in wasted medications. As you can see, it is important that public health gets to the hard work of teaching Americans to improve their health literacy skills to help control medical expenses as we simultaneously help people live longer.

Chapter 3: What is Health?

In the first few minutes of every presentation, I like to ask the questions, "What do you think health is?" and "Are you healthy?" Most people answer the first question with comments like, being able to do what you want, getting out of bed in a good mood, exercise, eating fruits and vegetables. In other words, we tend to think of health as a primarily physical thing with a bit of a mental health piece. There's more to it. According to the World Health Organization, health consists of physical, mental, social and spiritual health. We need to look closely at all four aspects of health.

Most people have a pretty good idea of what physical health encompasses. Physical health is why one would see a medical doctor. It includes illnesses and disabilities. Each of us is born with a certain health level and for the rest of our lives, we make decisions to, hopefully, help us stay that healthy or even get healthier. Exercise, enough sleep, good nutrition, avoiding bad habits, and learning to reduce stress are all included in the decisions made at home that reflect in the medical tests for issues like cholesterol, cancer, blood pressure and blood sugar levels. Young adults are most likely to only think physical health when they hear health.

Most people have a fairly straight forward understanding of mental health, too. Young adults tend to think of mental health as mental illness rather than health. This is slowly changing as advocates are in a national push to change the term from mental health to behavioral health. Behavioral health includes minor problems like anxiety and grief and a general outlook on life, up to more serious issues like learning disabilities, drug and alcohol addictions, schizophrenia, and Alzheimer's disease. At any time one's mental health can take a serious dive. For some people it can return to normal with a little bit of help, while others can be locked in a world of confusion that is hard to escape. One in four people will have a problem with their mental health at some point in their lives, but not all of the problems are long-term, chronic diseases.

One of the huge pieces of staying mentally healthy is to recognize that the stigma associated with mental illnesses is unfair to both the person who is struggling and their friends and family. Many young adults first develop serious mental health issues in their late teens and early 20s. There are lots of debates about why. I suspect some of this is a result of the extra stress young adults feel as they go to college or launch their careers. One of my favorite videos that explains mental health and stigma is on YouTube. You can find it under its title "If you have a brain, you have mental health" or by following this link (https://www.youtube.com/watch?v=oeWjqPb4o78&t=5s).

Social health is the aspect of health that as Americans, we often think about the least. It includes how we get along with others, as well as how others get along with us. The ability to hold a job, save for the future, make friends, raise a family, and enjoy the world are all aspects of social health. When physical health wanes in our old age, what keeps seniors happy and optimistic is their social health. Seeing their family and friends, living in a community with other seniors who are also socially healthy, having enough when they retire to make their lives easier, all offset the physical limitations of struggling to walk or hear or see as well. For young adults, financial planning for retirement, marriage or singleness, raising kids, holding down jobs, bullying vs boundaries on the job, relating to other generations, races, and cultures are all skills you will need to learn to be socially healthy.

Spiritual health is an area that we, as Americans, often do not discuss at all for fear of insulting others. Spiritual health is where one finds their inner strength to get through the bad moments of life. It is their personal beliefs that help them reach the end of their life feeling that they lead a purposeful life. It forms a core set of values on which people make decisions, including health choices.

Spiritual health and physical health decisions should work together to help people be at peace about what they are doing. No one should put their personal values to the side when making medical decisions. This is one of the crucial areas where health literacy training comes into place. If someone does not want to take a medication or get a blood transfusion because it violates their spiritual values, they need to be able to share that with their doctor in such a way, that the doctor looks for alternative ways to treat that patient. Choosing to raise a potentially ill child vs having an abortion is a real-world moment where young adults may have to balance their spiritual beliefs with medical advice. No doctor really knows how well a child will survive or thrive while they are in utero. Nor do they know how much the parents may learn about life, by accepting an ill child in their life. Most parents with kids with chronic illnesses could not imagine life without their child. This is not about ignoring the disease or being non-compliant. It is about balancing all aspects of your health.

When health literacy skills and all four aspects of health are taught to Americans, they have the potential to really change the way we handle life.

Chapter 4: Reading and Analyzing Medical Info

The first two skills in health literacy are the ability to read and write in English at a minimum of 8th grade level and the ability to analyze what you have read.

If you had learning disabilities that were ignored as a child, it is crucial that you go back and learn how to read smoothly. Adult education takes much more of a one-on-one approach to learning and there are a lot of different ways to both learn a skill and to teach it. Everyone can learn. Do not assume because you that because you did not do well growing up that you will also be unable to learn. I teach workforce development classes with students who often struggled through high school, and I promise that if you come with a good attitude, you can succeed.

The second health literacy skill is the ability to analyze what you have read. You should not only read the words on the page, but you should understand the deep meanings behind the words. Here is an example of what I mean. If I stand in the middle of the dog park and say, "That brown dog and that black dog are hers," how many people, at the minimum, are at the dog park? Think about it before you read the answer.

Did you say, one, two, three, four, or five? The answer is three. The person who is talking (me), the person I am talking to, and the "her" that owns the dogs. There may be other people there too, but the minimum is three.

Now let's up the difficulty of this. At minimum, how many dogs are at the dog park? Again take a few minutes and think about it before you read the next sentence.

The answer most people give is two. But the right answer is four. Had the sentence said "the black dog and the brown dog" two would have been correct. But when someone uses the word "that" dog, there must also be a "this" dog. So at the dog park there are currently (at least) two black dogs and two brown dogs. There may be a lot more dogs or dogs of other colors, but at minimum there are four dogs. Now, there is not a single word in that sentence that a first grade reader cannot read. And yet, the sentence stumps master's degree level English students all the time. This is the difference between being able to read and being able to analyze. Medical information is often more than the words. It is the analysis that makes it useful to our lives. This is one of the problems we have in health care. We can use easy words and still make the sentences impossible to understand.

To understand how the information applies to your health, let's try an example from the real world.

Almost everyone knows Dr. Oz from television. Every day he covers medical information with a real focus toward weight loss. Each day, he has some tip to help you lose a pound a week. He regularly gives five tips a week of "just do this and you can lose a pound a week." If you did all five things in a week, in theory, how much weight would you lose? Five pounds, right? In four weeks how much would you lose? 20 pounds! How about in 20 weeks? 100 pounds! How long before you totally disappeared?

Does weight lose really work like this? Maybe the first week. If you have 100 pounds or more to lose, maybe even the first 4 weeks, but after a while, it simply does not continue to work that way. And yet people will continue to try to use his easy solutions to weight loss instead of concentrating on what the medical world knows works—eat more fruits and veggies, drink more water, get enough sleep, and move 30 minutes a day. Knowing that you can use Dr. Oz's tips to kick start your weight loss journey, but you will have to do other things to continue to lose weight is a form of being able to analyze health care info.

In order to really be able to navigate the health care system well, especially if you use more holistic care, chiropractic care, or all natural supplements, you need to be able to understand what you are reading and hearing. Medical clinical trials require a lot of research and expense and the companies that chose to do that must meet strict double blind studies. They must report every weird side effect. If a patient dies during the trial (other than by accident or homicide) researchers must list death as a side effect. If researchers can prove the medication caused the death, it is unlikely the medication will ever reach consumers. They must run the drug or treatment through multiple levels of testings and the results must be the same over and over. A few years ago, the FDA even changed the way they allowed patents on new medications- a company must now prove the new medication is both safer and more effective than what is out on the market in order to get a patent.

For many homeopathic treatments, a single set of tests may be all they do and there is no oversight to prove the treatment works. Their clinical trial may simply be interviewing patients who have used the drugs. "I feel better" is not proof that the treatment made a difference. Now, that is not to say that homeopathic treatments don't make a difference, but it does mean that you cannot take the claim, "It's all natural, it won't hurt you" as the truth. Arsenic is all natural, but I would not want it in my food! It would kill me.

Understanding how to read and understand the extent of a study, or how to locate reliable information online are all so crucial to having excellent medical care. Being able to give your health symptoms to whoever is treating you in a clear concise manner is crucial to getting the right treatment. Whether that treatment comes from a doctor or your natural oils expert.

Chapter 5: Before You Seek Medical Care

Before you go to talk to your medical provider, you want to make sure you have written out your story. Your story goes back to your genetics, so anything you know about your parents and grandparents' health plus any serious chronic medical conditions your siblings have. Why? Because our genetics plus the way you were raised can influence your health now and into the future. In my family, we have no history of cancer, so I am not worried about early cancer screenings and I don't seek out care that includes preventing cancer. However, heart disease runs on both sides of my family, and both of my grandfathers died of heart attacks in their early 60s. I am much more concerned about getting early screenings for heart disease.

Jim Fixx wrote *The Complete Book of Running*, and was credited with helping start America's fitness craze in the 1970s. He started running to prevent dying early of a massive heart attack like his dad did at the age of 44. It shocked the running world in 1984, when Jim died of a massive heart attack at age 52. While running had helped delay the heart attack in his 40's, it only gave him eight more years of life over father. Because of Jim's story, medical personnel rely a lot more on genetics to determine how to help someone live a long time. Doctors check blood pressure, cholesterol, and triglycerides, which are all responses to some extent, the medical world's response to, "just because you can run a marathon, does not make you heart healthy."

Have your personal health history with you. List whether you had serious health issues in the past or are currently taking place in your life: surgeries, drug abuse, car accidents, sports injuries, domestic violence, child abuse, sexual abuse, poverty or hunger. Growing up with trauma can cause long-term health issues, so tell your providers this information, as well. Any prescribed medications, holistic treatments, essential oils, vitamins and over the counter medications, illegal drugs or alcohol you are taking need to be listed in your story. They can all impact how your body responds to a treatment or drug.

Additionally, explain why you are there today, symptoms you are having, how long they have been around, and what works and does not work to make it better.

Once you have your story written out, make sure you bring your health insurance card and a photo id to your doctor's appointments. Have three questions you need answered about your current condition. Make sure if you are in school or work that you understand if you need to miss work or school for a while, when you can return to work/school, and that the doctor writes it on a note.

If you struggle with a long-term, chronic illness or you are seeking treatment in an emergency room, you should try to bring someone over the age of 18 with you to be your advocate. This can be your parent, spouse, date, or best friend. Tell them on the way that they can speak up if they know something the doctor does not know, or if they have a question. This helps to ensure you have someone you can talk to at home who heard the doctor's instructions. If the two of you did not hear the instructions the same way, you can call back and confirm the directions.

Chapter 6: Medical Forms

When you get to the doctor's office, especially if it is a new doctor, you will be given a health history to fill out. Use the story you wrote out to answer all the questions. Make sure that anything on your written story is somewhere on that health form. Most doctors' offices are now equipped with patient portals that allow you to update info or email your doctor from your computer or phone. Sign up to use these patient portals. You may also want to find an app or website that will allow you to store your medical info.

You will also need to sign forms allowing the doctor to bill your insurance company. If you have health insurance, you certainly want them billed for your treatment. If you do not have insurance, the doctor's office may be able to suggest where you can get it. Each state now has an online website that allows you to enroll in health insurance. Trained enrollers can help you pick health insurance. Book Two of the Health Literacy Guides is all about choosing health insurance and understanding it better. It is a great follow-up book to this one.

You will also be given a form called HIPAA that guarantees the doctor will not share your medical info with others. But there may be people you are comfortable knowing your medical information or you would want them to know if you were in the hospital unconscious. Make sure that those people are listed on the exemption page. That page is not always given to you, but you should ask for it. Your parents, spouse or significant other, pastor, best friend, or siblings are some of the people you might list on the form. When my kids were little, their daycare provider was on both my form and theirs. If something happened to me while the kids were in the daycare's hands, I wanted their sitter to be able to have access to what was going on. If for some reason, I could not be reached in a medical emergency, I wanted their provider to have access to the ability to treat my child like they would their own. If you have a child with some sort of disability, your child's school principal or nurse might also be a possibility on the form. Make sure when you sign the notice that you got the HIPAA form, you have also added a couple of people to your exemption page.

If you live in New York State, you will also be asked about HIXNY (Health Insurance Exchange for New York). This is a medical records system for exchanging your health information between doctors, pharmacists, and hospitals. You want to sign YES to this form. Should you have a medical emergency, you want the hospital to be able to access your medical records from your doctors. You want them to know your latest medications. It could change the way they treat you. For instance, if you have a past history of drug addiction and you are involved in a car accident, you do not want them to give you a pain killer that will retrigger your drug addiction. If your primary doctor has your past drug abuse history in your records, the hospital will know too and can make a better decision for your overall health.

Every doctor's office has staff that can help you with the forms if you are confused. Just ask!

Chapter 7: Communicating with Your Provider

There are several key things you need to know about communicating with your provider. Again, whether you see a medical doctor, a physician assistant, a nurse, a chiropractor, or you prefer Reiki, vitamins, and essential oils, the ability to be clear about what is wrong will help you receive the right treatment. And it will help your holistic providers decide whether you might need a medical doctor. When I was 24, I worked for a company that packaged custom gifts based on nuts, fruit, and candy. Next door was my chiropractor. I called one day to say that I must have pulled a muscle lifting a box and could they see me because I had severe back pain. Fifteen minutes later, I was calling my primary care doctor; I actually had a kidney infection. Had I not been able to clearly tell my chiropractor about my back pain, he might have tried treating my back pain, instead of recognizing that what I needed was an antibiotic (and a lecture on drinking more water in the heat of the summer.)

In order to communicate with your doctor, you must know how to:

1. Clearly and concisely list all symptoms both new and old.
2. Remind your doctor of pre-existing medical conditions.
3. List all medications you take (no matter where you get them).
4. Be patient as he asks questions. Listen closely to what he is asking. He is seeking information from you without trying to put words in your mouth.
5. Use the right words. "It hurts" is not enough. These are some of the words that can mean or describe pain—burns, itches, constant, periodic, throbs, aches, dull, or sharp.
6. Be able to tell exactly where it hurts. "I have a headache" is a great start. But is it the back of your head: most likely a tension based headache or might even come from a neck or shoulder injury. The front of your head around your eyes and nose—likely a sinus problem.

Does the pain focus on only the left or right side of your head: this is more likely to be a migraine. Each are treated very differently. The same thing with stomach pain—coming from the stomach, gallbladder, from your appendix, uterine cramps for women, bladder area. On your foot—your toes, arches, or ankle area, along with the top and bottom of your foot. The more specific you can be, the faster and easier it is to get the right diagnosis.

7. If you have a chronic medical condition, especially if you see different doctors or you use a combo of holistic and western medicine, you may want to keep a notebook of all you are doing to treat it. You may also want to bring a friend/family member with you to help ensure you understand the doctor thoroughly. The Emergency Room is the one place I highly recommend you never leave without having a friend listen to the discharge directions. You will almost always leave with a new diagnosis and treatment after waiting hours and being in pain. It is so easy to leave the ER without really

understanding what is going on with your body. Make sure someone is there when you leave to help you get all the info you need.

8. Once you give the doctor all the info you have, you need to be able to make sure you understand what he is telling you. The Teach Back Method is a great way to do that.

The "teach back method" was originally created by the medical system to make sure the patient understood the doctor. It takes about three to four minutes to do and you literally "teach back" to the doctor or nurse everything you learned during the appointment. You can do this or if you have a friend going with you, he can. It gives the doctor a chance to correct any information that you have wrong or for the doctor to further explain something to you that you may be confused about. (This is also a good tool for bosses and spouses).

To use the method, you wait until the end of the appointment then say, "When I get home, my mom/boyfriend/bff will ask what happened at the doctor's office today. If I tell them this _______________ (fill in the blank with what you think happened in the office), will I have missed any crucial information? Your doctor should be able to tell you, "yes you have that all right," "you have most of it right, but this part," or "no, let's go over it all again." If the doctor has to re-explain you anything, you should re-teach the doctor again until his answer is "yes, you have this all right."

On the next page, you will find a diagram of the teach back method.

The Teach Back Method

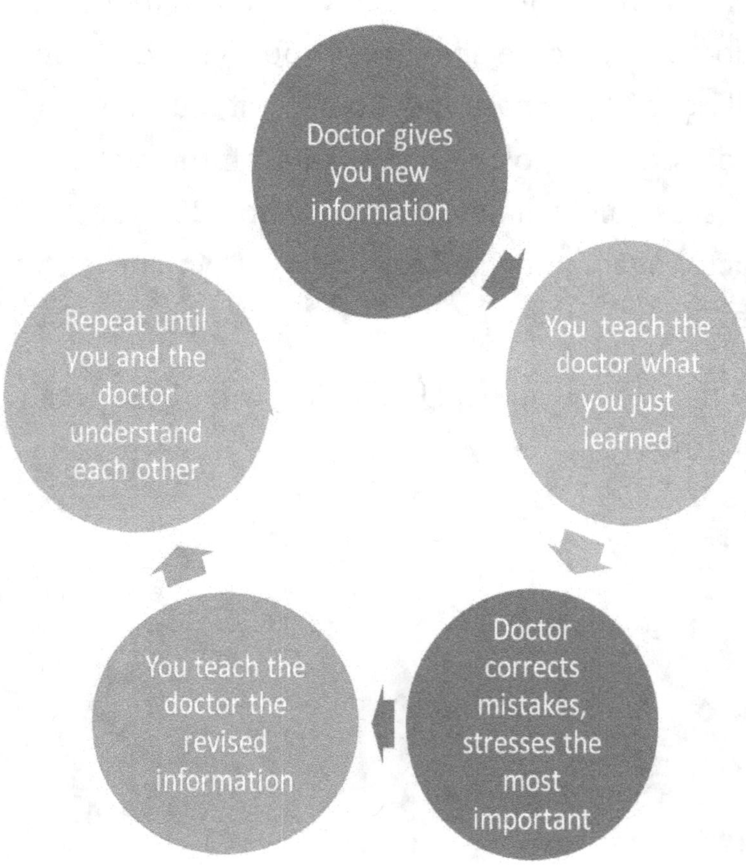

Chapter 8: Choosing a Treatment

Most times doctors are going to say, "this is what is wrong; this is how you fix it." For some things, like high blood pressure or being overweight, you may want to try a holistic treatment before you do medication. However, there are also times when you have an illness with choices for treatments. How do you choose?

1. Be informed.
    a. Know what happens if you choose not to do anything to treat your medical problem. (Lots of people ignore their illnesses, which has the effect of choosing to do nothing.)
    b. If you prefer a holistic way to treat it, be prepared to share that with your medical provider. You have the right to try treating yourself with essential oils, or visiting a chiropractor, or walking more, but you must have a way to follow up

with your doctor or nurse to ensure your non-traditional system is working.

c. Understand all the medical options. Research other medications and treatments plans using webmd.com, pubmed.com, or cdc.gov. Call a local telemedicine company or ask your doctor or insurance company for a second opinion.

2. Be honest. Tell your doctor about your lifestyle and values that may impact your treatment options. If you have a strong faith and believe that God can heal you or you aren't allowed blood products, share that with your doctor. If you have a fear about the treatment, you have someone in your family that tried that option and it didn't work, or you just can't see yourself doing all the follow up, let the doctor know that. Balancing your mental, spiritual or social health must be balanced with your physical health.

3. Be realistic—if you know from the start you won't follow a treatment plan, share that with

your provider. Give him a chance to find an alternative.

4. Be consistent—if you start a treatment and find that you cannot follow the plan, tell your doctor immediately.

Some of the areas where these issues may come into play for a young adult could come in areas like sexual lifestyles, cancer treatments, unplanned pregnancies and abortions, treating obesity, and stopping smoking or other bad habits. The better you know yourself, the better the provider caring for you can match your treatment to you.

Chapter 9: Medications

Let's play a little game called "What is the Drug?"

To reduce nausea:
- Ginger tea bought at a health food store
- Anti-nausea liquid bought at a pharmacy
- Marijuana bought on the street corner

To reduce anxiety:
- St John's Wort (an herb) bought from the chiropractor
- Prescription from your doctor
- A glass of wine

To sooth a rash:
- Lotion bought through a cosmetics company
- Vitamin recommended by your personal trainer
- Oatmeal soak suggested by your doctor

Did you guess they all are drugs? A good functional definition of **medication** is "ANYTHING you put in or on your body to treat a symptom, change the way you feel or improve your health, no matter where you get it from."

It is important that you understand that anything that you take to feel better is a medication and needs to be recorded in your medical records. The vitamins, essential oils, over the counter or illegal drugs, herbal supplements you take may interfere with each other or create side effects.

Here are the side effects to the holistic options listed above. Ginger: too much causes diarrhea, mouth irritation, heartburn, bloating, flatulence, upset stomach and possible sedation. St John's Wort: overdose can cause fever, difficulty walking, hallucinations, and a rapid heart rate. Oatmeal baths: those with Celiac's disease can react to the oatmeal and bathing for more than 10-20 minutes at a time can make rashes worse. These side effects can be as serious as the side effects of a traditional prescribed medication.

The good news is as we learn more about drug interactions and side effects, the medical records are able to keep up. So as long as you are putting all your medications into your medical history, the doctors and pharmacists you see will get a warning from the computer systems when a new drug is prescribed. And you will probably notice that more and more doctors will suggest vitamins, probiotics, and other non-traditional medications to treat certain conditions.

Side effects are effects of a medication on the human body that are not the planned reaction. Sometimes side effects are not a problem to you. Occasionally, a drug is given for both its original purpose and its side effects. When a drug's side effects are pretty consistent, it is sometimes prescribed for its side effect alone. Right now, one of my kids is having trouble sleeping and her anxiety is high. Many of the traditional sleeping medications would interfere with her anti-anxiety meds. So she was given a muscle relaxant that's side effect is it makes people sleepy. Side effects are not always a bad thing. But it is possible that a drug's side effects annoy you or create a symptom that is actually dangerous. Be sure to discuss any issues you think have been caused by a medication with your pharmacists.

There are 13,000 known ways for the body to go wrong, 6000 treatments and 4000 medications. Doctors know about the illnesses that can go wrong with your body. Pharmacists know all the medications. Let me say that again—doctors know about illnesses; pharmacists know the medications. Pharmacists are the professionals you want to talk to when your drugs are an issue. They know what medications work similarly in your body and what will create the same dangerous or annoying side effect. They can call your doctor for you and explain why a different drug would work just as well, and they can help you get the best medication for yourself.

One of the biggest mistakes people make when taking a medication is taking the right medication for the wrong reason. There are three reasons a person is given a drug: to treat a symptom, a short-term illness or to manage a chronic (lifelong) illness. In America, we take most over the counter medications to treat symptoms. Have a headache, take a Tylenol. Have a cough, take cough medicine. When the headache or the cough is gone, you stop taking the drug, which is a great plan if you have a simple symptom.

When you are treating a short-term illness like strep throat, you are often given a drug that requires you take all the medication and not stop when the symptom (the sore throat) is gone. Usually these medications come with no refills, but a strict direction from the doctor and on the bottle to use all the medication. If you do not take it all, you risk not killing off all the germs and having a repeat of the infection that is even harder to treat.

When you treat a chronic illness, the medication is usually given with refills. It is anticipated that you will take the medication for the rest of your life and you will be refilling your medication every month in the local drug store or sometimes every three months by mail. There are times when a chronic illness can go away, and one can come off the medication. For instance, a type 2 diabetic who loses weight and learns to eat better, may be able to come off their drugs that helped control their blood sugar levels. But you should not come off any medication that treats a chronic illness without your doctor's preapproval and monitoring your body for reactions.

Mental health medications are one of the types of drugs that are most often used wrong. Patients often struggle with side effects and it can take lots of different attempts at dosage levels and different medication combinations before the patient feels better. Unfortunately, when they feel better they decide that now that they feel good, they do not need the drugs anymore. The patient will stop taking the drug, but because it has built up in their body and they feel stable. It will take a few weeks for the patient to start to feel the illness come back. By then, the patient often misses the connection between coming off the medication a few weeks ago and their cruddy feelings now. It may take them a few more weeks before they seek medical care and proper meds again. By now, they often have to start with lower doses, built up the drugs in their body again, and get stabilized. All of this un-medicated time can be dangerous to a person's mental health. And it comes from the misunderstanding that the patient has that once the symptoms of his illness are gone, he does not need his medication any more.

Chapter 10: Healthy Behaviors

In 1972, researchers identified seven behaviors that indicated someone was living a healthy lifestyle: getting 7-8 hours of sleep, not smoking, eating breakfast, regular exercise, not having more than 1 alcoholic drink a day for women or 2 for men, not eating between meals (not eating over your calorie range), and not being more than 10% overweight. We are going to go over these really quickly.

SLEEP

Sleep is THE biggest issue for most young adults. Studying, odd work hours, taking on the stresses of growing up, and parties all interfere with getting solid sleep. When you do not sleep enough, there are serious health consequences.

Sleep allows your brain to regenerate brain cells and process what you have learned during the day. Students who get enough sleep move the things they learned that day from their short-term memory to their long-term memory. That means less studying later, because the info they learn is now stored where they can access it for midterms and finals.

Short-term problems with lack of sleep also include lack of alertness, impaired long-term and short-term memory, relationship stress and impatience, a greater likelihood for car accidents.

Long-term problems that go with lack of sleep includes high blood pressure, diabetes, heart attacks, strokes, depression, poor choices, obesity, and lower sex drive. Dark circles under eyes and premature skin wrinkling can make it physically obvious that you are sleep deprived. An increase in cortisol (the fight or flight hormone) shuts down your ability to think clearly and breaks down collagen making you more susceptible to sprains and strains. Do your best to get 7-8 hours of sleep each night.

NOT SMOKING

I am not sure there is a single thing I can say about the dangers of smoking tobacco that you all don't already know. Smoking is tied to activation in your body of every known cancer. It makes every chronic illness worse. While it may make you think you have calmed yourself with the cigarette, your body is really internally struggling with oxygen and carbon dioxide levels. Smoking lowers your immune system, making it easier to get colds, flus, and other illnesses.

If you have not smoked, please don't start. E-cigarettes and vaping, originally designed as stop smoking options, are healthier than tobacco if you are looking to quit, but they have their own health risks. Most of the e-cigs and vape products have been bought out by the cigarette companies who immediately began tampering with the chemicals to make them more addicting. If you don't use them, don't start. But if you smoke tobacco, they can be used safely as a step down before you quit smoking everything.

When you want to stop smoking, there are lots of ways to try. It takes the average smoker 7 times to permanently quit. Relapses (picking up a cigarette after stopping for more than a week) are totally normal. If you see that cigarette as a relapse instead of sign it is too difficult, it is easier to not pick up the next one.

Cravings themselves only last in your brain for three minutes and most cravings are over in the first week to ten days. Make a list of things you can do for three minutes to avoid the cravings: use hand lotion, sing a song, call a friend, make a list of things you for which you're grateful. During the first day or two, the cravings may come back quickly, but after that, your body usually sends out cravings tied to what you are doing socially. Having a drink of coffee or alcohol will often trigger a craving, or driving in your car where you smoked will make you want a smoke. Try new things—new ways to drink your coffee, try a new brand of beer, drive a different way to work or school—that are easy ways to avoid these cue driven cravings.

Medications may help. While there are stop smoking meds, you may find that anti-anxiety meds or ADHD meds may help if you were smoking to calm anxieties or help you focus. Drinking lots of water (64-120 oz) a day can flush the toxins out of your body and help minimize cravings. Another trick is to buy a new brand. Most people do not like new brands and will decide that it is worth it to quit over forcing yourself to smoke a brand you don't like.

EATING BREAKFAST

Not eating breakfast seems like such a small detail, yet in the scheme of healthy eating and staying within your recommended calories, eating something healthy within a half hour of getting up kick starts your metabolism, leaves you less hungry at lunch, and allows you to continue to make good food choices for the rest of the day.

Eating breakfast should not be thought of as a couple of donuts or some high sugared pastry or muffin. Even first thing in the morning, your body wants fiber, protein, vitamins and minerals. Protein and veggie/fruit shakes are a healthy option if that appeals to you. High fiber breakfast bars without a lot of fat and salt are good options for an on-the-go meal. Cottage cheese and fruit, yogurt and fruit, nuts or nut butters with veggies, eggs with veggies cooked into them, all meet the fiber/protein plus fruits or veggies combo that most people need to stay healthy. Cereal is often too carb loaded to stick with your body through the morning, although there are some of them that are great. An ounce of cheese and some grapes is my daughter's favorite grab and go breakfast. Even a slice of leftover veggie pizza from the night before may be a healthier breakfast option than many cereals. Make sure you have also had 1 to 2 (8 ounce) glasses of water by the time you finish breakfast. Dehydration is a dangerous way to go through the day.

REGULAR EXERCISE

There is probably little I can really tell you about the need for regular exercise that you haven't already heard. But I still need to cover this a bit.

Exercise is just movement at a speed that challenges your brain, heart, lungs, and muscles to keep up. For cardio exercises (those exercises that use a lot of oxygen in your muscles) you need a minimum of 30 minutes a day, 5 days a week. The workouts can be done in as little as 10 minutes, 3 times a day. An easy way to test if you are working hard enough during a cardio workout is you should not *want* to talk to a person next to you, but you can.

Muscle building should also be part of your weekly exercises. A couple of times a week with weights, pull-ups or pushups, yoga, and other forms of exercise that strengthen your muscles are necessary. The more muscle mass your body has, the faster it burns through calories.

As Americans, we tend to take an all or nothing option towards life. I am always amazed at how many people don't exercise because they cannot figure out how to find the time to exercise. But your body is better off if you do 10 minutes worth of cardio a few days a week and 2 minutes of muscle building exercises a few days a week, then none at all. And as you start finding a few minutes here and there and feeling better, it will make it easier to find a few more minutes in your life for more.

ONE OR TWO GLASSES OF ALCOHOL

First of all, let's remember that alcohol in the US is only legal for those over 21, unless given to them by a parent. And many people have a family history of drug and alcohol abuse, so for those youths, even one drink a day could be harmful. Again, I remind you that your physical health choices should never compromise your spiritual health choices, so if your faith does not believe in drinking alcohol, please do not do so.

For those who chose to drink, one glass per day, no more than four per week is considered by most researchers a safe level of alcohol consumption for most women. Men, who typically have more muscle mass than women can handle up to two glasses a day, with their upper limit at about seven a week. This is not a goal to be reached, but a maximum not to exceed. And in no way does this guarantee you won't develop an alcohol problem. My firm rule is if I want a drink, I can have one. If I need a drink, I should never touch it.

There are some proven health benefits to some alcohols. One glass of red wine (4 ounces) daily has benefits to those with heart disease and stroke risks. One glass of beer a day (12 ounces) reduces the risk for kidney stones. But again I warn that you have plenty of time in health to start with a glass a day of alcohol for your health and you risk so much if you develop a drinking problem, that I want to you be very wary of using "it's healthy" as an excuse to be unhealthy.

NOT EATING BETWEEN MEALS

This is by far one of the most controversial of the suggestions. Many people find that grazing their way through the day instead of three big meals makes it easier for them to eat the right amount of calories and nutrition.

There are many places on the web where you can type in your height and weight and get recommended calorie counts for yourself. Here is one of them https://my-calorie-counter .com/calorie-calculator/. Another option if you want ideas and a way to track what you eat is SparkPeople.com or SparkTeen.com.

In general, there are a couple of "tricks" to eating healthy. First is to drink plenty of water- at least 64oz (4 disposable 16.9 ounces bottles of water) and potentially more. Your body cannot tell the difference between mild hunger and mild thirst, so always assuming thirst is the issue first, helps to curb overeating. Second, chew your food slowly and try to eat somewhere where it is pleasant and enjoyable to eat slowly. This gives your stomach time to get full and tell your brain. Never have seconds until 20 minutes after you have finished your firsts. Most of the time, you will find you are full.

Third, aim for lots of fruits and vegetables in your meals. The current recommendation is five to seven servings a day and there is a push to go to seven to nine servings. In general, if you are putting food into your mouth, you should be eating a fruit or vegetable along with whatever else you are eating. And finally, track what you are eating. It truly helps you "see" what you are doing well and where you need help.

NOT BEING MORE THAN 10 % OVERWEIGHT

Using the above websites or Webmd.com can help you find out if you are more than 10% overweight. Because Americans are struggling not only with being overweight but being obese, we have lost our natural ability to look at ourselves and our friends, and judge whether our weight is ok. Most people I meet who are 20% overweight believe they are at a healthy weight. If you are more than 10% overweight, please consider losing some weight.

Chapter 11: Behavioral Health

Behavioral health is the new word for mental health, learning disabilities, as well as drug and alcohol addictions. While 1 in 10 people can manage their physical health well, only 1 in 33 can handle their mental health well. One of the biggest problems we have with treating behavioral health issues is stigma. Stigma is a attitude of disgrace over a particular illness or condition. If your doctor told you that you had cancer, you would seek treatment, ask for help, and share that info with your school and friends so they understood what was happening with you. If your doctor says you have anxiety, you will probably ignore it. If a school diagnoses a child with a learning disability, many parents will blame the school district or teacher that their child is struggling. They may not share with the school what is happening at home because they do not want their child "labeled." You may take this same attitude as you go into college or a job. But hiding a diagnosis does not make it go away, it just prevents people who could help you with it from giving you a hand.

Drug and alcohol addictions are similar. The more you share your struggles, the more support you should find for succeeding despite your problems. Nobody is interested in picking on you for your health history—physical or behavioral. Share your story and allow the world to support you. Share your story and others can share theirs. This is a core basis of AA, NA, or Celebrate Recovery: to use social health and friendships to help you overcome your addictions to anything.

As young people stop living with their parents, take on more responsibility, and make choices for themselves, they automatically increase the stress in their life. For many people, this extra stress triggers many forms of mental illnesses. Depression, Schizophrenia, Bipolar disorder are often diagnosed for the first time in young adults. Mental health meds, unlike physical health meds, can take weeks to build up in one's system before they are effective. It often takes repeated attempts at different doses or different meds to find a treatment that truly helps you continue to function in the world. Don't give up. Keep trying until you find a medication that allows you to enjoy life and learning again.

Do not be afraid to seek counseling through a therapist or a small group. Certain things are easier to talk through with a professional. Denial does not help anyone. If you know someone that you suspect has a mental health problem, talk to them. Encourage them to see a someone who can help. Often their primary care doctor is the best place to start. But if you think they are at real risk of harm to themselves or others, take them to an emergency room. Be the person who can help save someone else's life.

Chapter 12: Pain, Pleasure and Drugs

Pain happens when nerves in your body are triggered by pressure or chemicals. When these nerves are activated your brain responds to the concept of pain. The amount of pain you feel is based on how frequently those nerves send their messages to the brain as well as how many nerves are sending the messages. When your brain thinks "the body is in pain" it releases dopamine to slow down or stop the pain signals.

When you are hurt or after surgery, you will be given the mildest pain medication that has been proven to eliminate pain from that "injury" (surgery or damage). The medication may be based on what the injury is, how extensive it is or how many pain nerves are in that location of your body. Most people need to take that pain medication for at least a few days. When you body is in pain, the brain and the chemical systems move to fight or flight and do not heal your body or activate the immune system as quickly as when you are pain free. Therefore, it is important for a quick recovery to use pain medications to control the pain while you heal. Using the least amount and the weakest pain drug that still works to eliminate pain is good. But "toughing it out," and "it's not that bad" are attitudes that cause your body to take longer to heal as well as raise your risk of infection. Once you have stopped taking an opioid for pain relief, you should not restart or take it for a new injury. Use wet coffee grounds to neutralize the rest of the pills and turn them in on a medication take back event. (Call your local hospital, pharmacy or sheriff's office to find out where they are held in your community)

Pleasure occurs when the nerves in your body tell your brain something nice is going on outside your body. Endorphins (body chemicals) are released in your body as a response to mild stress, exercise, sex, and other pleasurable moments. Your brain senses those nerves and chemicals as "FUN!!!!" Dopamine and serotonin are the endorphins that are triggered during pleasurable activities. Technically, the only two things you really enjoy are serotonin and dopamine. Low serotonin levels are responsible for some people's depression, as they chemically cannot feel "fun or happiness."

Wait, did I just say dopamine is a pleasure chemical? And that it is a pain relief chemical? Yes! Dopamine both shuts down the pain center and rewards the pleasure center of the brain. Dopamine is very similar chemically to morphine, heroin, codeine, and other opioids. Which is why these drugs are so excellent as pain killers. Because when taken, they both shut down the pain center and activate the pleasure center. This duality is why people can easily become addicted to opioids but not other pain killers like ibuprofen (Motrin) or acetaminophen (Tylenol.)

Opioid receptors (the locations in your body that respond to dopamine and other opioids are found in the brain, spinal cord, and the digestive system. We know that there are three major receptor types and scientists are studying on mice how these receptors work win relationship to pain and pleasure. If we can find a medication that relieves the pain without triggering the pleasure centers, we believe we can lessen the likelihood of people becoming addicted when given these pain meds.

Tolerance is another factor in the addiction cycle. Tolerance is the body's ability to accept or reject the action of a drug, poison or other chemical. Many drugs are not affected by tolerance. For instance, most high blood pressure medications can be taken for years without needing an increase in the medication for it to continue working. But opioids are a classification of medications in which the body can build up a tolerance for them- in other words, the longer you take an opioid the less affect it works. In which case, you need more of the medication for it to work well in your body. This biochemical need for more of the drug is what pushes misusers of opioids into full blown addicts.

Opioids also have a unique reaction in your body once it is out of your system for about 72 hours. Your tolerance level goes back down to that of someone who hadn't used the drug. While this is excellent for someone who has been given the drug for temporary pain management and then needs it again in a few years for another incident, it can be a real hazard for someone abusing the drugs.

When someone smokes cigarettes at a pack a day and then stops smoking, tolerance is not a factor. They can restart smoking at a cigarette a day or a pack a day and it won't change the effect it has on the body. However, when someone stops using an opioid and starts again, the amount they ingest can be deadly. Let's use the example of someone who is abusing codeine pills. They started taking one pill and when that was no longer effective, they moved to two pills. Depending on a long they have been using the pills, they may be up to 4,7 or 10 pills at a time. Then they decide to quit, end up in rehab or jail, or for some reason stop using for a few days. If they restart, they are not likely to start with 1 pill again, although their body would only need that amount to get high. Instead they will start with the same or almost the same amount they ended with. Since their body doesn't need that level to get high, the drug will now overwhelm their system and they are likely to overdose and die.

There are several risk factors involved in becoming addicted and overdosing. Genetics, loss of tolerance, mixing drugs, using alone, variations in drug strength and purity, serious illness, depression, unstable housing, injecting the opioids, or a history of a previous overdoses. Genetics, illnesses, and depression is something that one cannot do a lot about. Variations in drug strength and mixing drugs can easily happen when one gets his drugs illegally from anyone who has them. Using drugs alone and injecting drugs should be a huge warning sign one needs help. Lose of tolerance means if someone stops and restarts, he needs to know enough to restart at a lower level. Once one has become addicted, the likelihood of unstable housing and a history of overdoses is likely to result in death as well. If you suspect someone is abusing drugs, speak up and offer to help them get care. Drugs do not make people fall asleep. The brain and body are shutting down in reaction to the drugs. If you think they could be overdosing, call 911.

For those who struggle with chronic pain, there are other things that can help manage the pain. On New York's capital region, the Saratoga Hospital has a pain management clinic that can help people who struggle with pain. Chiropractic care, therapeutic massage, acupuncture and acupressure are all great ways to get pain relieve in some circumstances. Over the counter medications, herbal remedies and essential oils may help to relieve pain rather than using an opioid medication. Meditation, deep breathing, slow stretching like tai-chi or yoga may also lessen pain. Using heat or cold can also help. Often doctors will suggest starting with cold to reduce swelling and then using heat later to increase blood flow to the area. Some people do well alternating the two. When I had surgery on my knees and was doing physical therapy, I found cold on the knee caps and heat on the back of my knees at the same time worked best. Diet and good hydration (drinking lots of water) can also improve pain levels. When your body is healing it needs more protein and micronutrients from fruits and vegetables. The tendency to say, "I'm in pain and I want chocolate, Doritos, ice cream, etc." needs to be replaced by the attitude of "In order for my body to heal, I need fruits, vegetables, and protein (meat, nuts, cheese, etc.)"

Releasing more dopamine naturally also helps. Physically, repetitive motions like rocking, dancing, knitting and casting for fish works. Use your senses to trigger pleasant experiences or memories, taste a favorite food or use aromatherapy to smell something you love. Use music or sound machines to relax you. Massages, holding hands, and hugging all release dopamine. Looking at family photos or other things you love can also help.

Mentally, you can express gratitude to the people around you, add laughter to your life, or just insist you are going to have a positive attitude really helps as well. Socially, going out with friends, playing games or practicing random acts of kindness are all proven pain killers. Spiritually, going to church, temple or gathering with others who share your values, praying, and seeking forgiveness all release stress and add to natural pain relief. Many people living in chronic pain do these things and comment that they get a placebo effect from enjoying life instead of focusing on the pain. But it's not a placebo effect. You are feeling pleasure which releases dopamine. And the dopamine also eases the pain.

Chapter 13: Depression and Suicide

One in four people will struggle with some form of mental health problem in their life. They may go through a tough time in their life and have anxiety. Maybe their friend dies, they can't get over it, and develop complicated grief. Learning disabilities like ADHD, autism or Alzheimer's disease are all mental health issues that can last a longer time. Depression is likely to build slowly or can come on quickly and either way can lead to suicide.

Suicide is the 10th leading cause of death in the US. And the second leading cause of death in college students. Keeping up grades, isolation from friends and family, and the responsibilities of growing up can add to a feeling of being overwhelmed. A history of mild depression at a younger age and lack of a good support system are two of the strongest predicators of suicidal thoughts and actions in young adults. Growing up in a home with domestic violence or with a mother that struggled with depression are two other suicide risk factors. Not sleeping, sleeping too much, not eating, and being "no fun" are all signs of depression. Studies show that simply thinking about suicide was not actually a predictor of attempting suicide. Making a plan, however, was. Two in ten college students who attempted suicide did not think about it in the days before they tried it.

Some of the best ways to prevent suicide are to have friends, to be connected to the college community, and to be willing to seek treatment. Suicide and depression are definitely two areas where stigma often prevents depressed people from asking about help and their loved ones and friends from asking how they are feeling. If your friend has a cold, you may offer Nyquil or at least ask how they are feeling. Yet we get hints of sadness or stress and we ignore it, not wanting to get "in their business." The best thing you can do for a friend who seems depressed or even suicidal is to ask the questions. Are you sad? Have you thought about suicide? And if they answer yes, "how can I help?" or "will you promise to stay alive until we can you take you somewhere to talk to someone professional?" Like an overdose, if their symptoms are severe, the best thing to do is call 911.

In Conclusion

This book is meant to be a brief overview of healthy living and talking to your doctor. Every chapter here could be a full book or two. Do not hesitate to research for yourself anything you need more information about. You may find what you are looking for in other *Health Literacy Guide* books or by Googling the topics. There is always more to learn about any given topic. Then you still have to take what you have learned and apply that information to your life. Strawberries are a great healthy food, unless you are personally allergic to it. You cannot make health decisions for your life based on other people's decisions. You must know about your own body and your own health history. Health Literacy is all about not only knowing the info, but using it well to keep yourself alive and well.

Additional Books by Karen Laing

All books are available on Amazon.com on either Kindle or in paperback.

If you are interested in ordering large quantities for your business, church, or organization, you can reach the author at info@healthliteracyforall.org. Put "Large Book Order" in the email. For large discounted quantities please be aware that the shipping time can take three weeks, so plan ahead.

Book Titles

Health Literacy Guide Series

Aging with Style

If you are a senior, love a senior, or hope to be a senior someday, this book is for you. We will take a health and wellness look at the hard questions in the aging process...Where will you live? Can you communicate well with your doctor and family? What about driving and senior fraud? These and other topics covered. Use this book as a catalyst for having these hard discussions with your family members.

Picking Health Insurance

Understanding the basics of health insurance gets more complicated every year. This book is designed to cover what health insurance is, how to use it well, and what things you should look at when you compare coverages. This book is a basics class so it works whether you are picking from your state's health exchange, from your employer, or Medicare. Additional information includes national resources on finding low-cost help and understanding a bit about the basics of Medicare.

Stress: The Good, the Bad, the Ugly

We all think that stress is "bad" for our health. But did you know that you couldn't survive without some stress in your life. Your body thrives on it! On the other hand, chronic stress can have long-term health complications and can make many diseases impossible to successfully treat. Come learn more about how stress impacts health and how to lessen the bad kinds of stress in your life.

Teens and Young Adults

When HIPAA was signed into law, adults were given the promise that no one else would have access to their medical records without their full knowledge and consent. While that was great for adults, it often leaves teens turning 18 in a position to have to navigate the health care system without their parents' help any longer. Because our medical system insists parents are active in their teen's health concerns until the day they turn 18, and then they cannot have access to their kid's records, it can leave teens unprepared to cope. This book teaches teens on how to begin taking charge and gives the 18+ young adult key skills to navigate the health care system alone.

Raising Health Literate Kids

In order to avoid having your child turn 18 and not know how to talk to their doctor, fill out medical forms, or make health decisions on their own, the child needs to be taught from a young age. This guide helps parents with kids as young as 2 begin the process of teaching their children to speak up for themselves, ask questions, and gain other crucial health literacy skills. Many of these skills can be easily transferred to schooling, work and social situations as well. Help your child learn more than just their ABC's and 123's. Help them learn to be healthy for life.

Spiritually Able: Help Your Place of Worship Integrate the Disabled with Ease

Every house of worship I have ever been in wants their members to feel like a family and participate fully in the life of the community. It is an integral part of having spiritual health. Yet often we ignore those who have physical, mental, or social health limitations. This book is designed to help your place of worship work alongside other houses of worship to not only care for the needs of the disabled within your community but get them actively serving too.

The Everyday Christian's Guides

Prayer

Whether you are new to talking directly to God, you have just run out of things to say, or you feel like no one is listening, this book can help take you from where you are to a closer walk with God. Also available in Spanish and French.

Spiritual Warfare

We start with the verse, "If God is for you, who can be against you?" and take a closer look at who gets in our way of having a great relationship with God. We also look at what it means to put on "the whole armor of God" and the concept "the weapons of our warfare are not earthly." See how the book of Ephesians takes us on a journey of training for war. Soon to be available in French.

Health and Healing

God's view of health and healing from a total look at health—physical, mental, social and spiritual. This book also covers miraculous healings, allowing God to be your strength through illness, and death as the ultimate healing. Soon to be available in Spanish.

Bible Study

The Bible is GOD's set of directions for a good life on earth. It is full of laws, suggestions, and hints to help us not only survive on earth but to thrive. It is also the greatest love story ever told. Christians are told they need to read the Bible. There are thousands of Bible Study books that help us learn what is in there. This book explains more of why you would want to pick up your Bible daily or open the app on your phone! And if the entire process seems overwhelming, there are tips and tricks to get started and to stay motivated. Come read how much GOD loves you.

Forgiveness

Forgiveness is an idea born from the intense love of GOD for his creation. It is a concept that is often misunderstood, misinterpreted or worse, misapplied. It is a hard thing to understand and harder to do.

Especially when the pain is deep, and the person doesn't "deserve" to be forgiven. But it is what we are called to do, and this book will help you understand why GOD feels this is so important as well as how we can forgive.

****

And as always, if you have received valuable tips and training out of our books, we would love you to make a comment on Facebook, at HealthLiteracyForAll.org, on LinkedIn at Karen Burhans Laing, or on Amazon.com. Even better, copy and paste your comment to them all! Of course the ultimate compliment is to buy another book for a friend!

Be Healthy!

Karen

www.ingramcontent.com/pod-product-compliance
Lightning Source LLC
Chambersburg PA
CBHW061726250726
48657CB00002B/799